Grateful
FOR
Grace

Grateful FOR Grace

Reflections on Caring for Mom

by Donna Olivia

XULON PRESS

Xulon Press
2301 Lucien Way #415
Maitland, FL 32751
407.339.4217
www.xulonpress.com

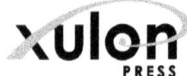

© 2021 by Donna Olivia

All rights reserved solely by the author. The author guarantees all contents are original and do not infringe upon the legal rights of any other person or work. No part of this book may be reproduced in any form without the permission of the author. The views expressed in this book are not necessarily those of the publisher.

Due to the changing nature of the Internet, if there are any web addresses, links, or URLs included in this manuscript, these may have been altered and may no longer be accessible. The views and opinions shared in this book belong solely to the author and do not necessarily reflect those of the publisher. The publisher therefore disclaims responsibility for the views or opinions expressed within the work.

Unless otherwise indicated, Scripture quotations taken from the New King James Version (NKJV). Copyright © 1982 by Thomas Nelson, Inc. Used by permission. All rights reserved.

Paperback ISBN-13: 9781662815980
Ebook ISBN-13: 9781662815997

Dedication

This book is dedicated to our matriarch, Ms. Grace who brought us through difficult times, disciplined us when necessary, taught us the importance of education and the arts, and instilled values in us through God's loving Grace.

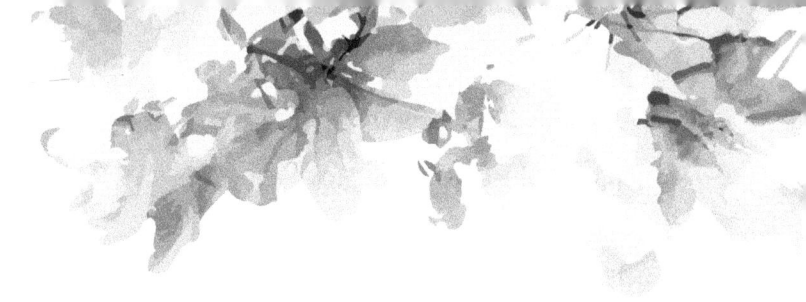

Table of Contents

Preface ix
Chapter 1. Growing Up with Grace. 1
Chapter 2. Mom Lives with Me Now 7
Chapter 3. Feeding Time 11
Chapter 4. Brushing Mom's Hair. 15
Chapter 5. Hats, Lots and Lots of Hats! . . . 18
Chapter 6. Mom's Wise Words
               (Grace-isms) 22
Chapter 7. Struggling with Memory 25
Chapter 8. The Blessed Decision 29
Chapter 9. Mom's Reflections
               (Teaching Still) 33
Chapter 10. Getting Me through School . 37
Chapter 11. A Little More Time Together. . 41
Chapter 12. Taking Mom Out 44
Chapter 13. Never Say Never. 48
Chapter 14. I Wondered, I Waited
                (and Tried Not to Worry). 52

Grateful for *Grace*

Chapter 15. The New Normal............ 56
Chapter 16. You Are Not Alone 60
Chapter 17. God's Grace............... 64
Chapter 18. Caring for Mom as a Work of HeART 67
Chapter 19. The Little Things 71
Chapter 20. Emotional Moments........ 76
Chapter 21. Care for the Caregiver 82
Chapter 22. Just Thankful 86
Summary............................. 90

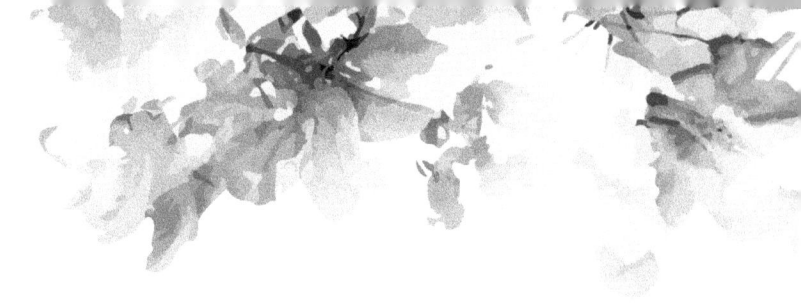

Preface

Caring for a loved one is such a rewarding experience, despite the concerns for their well-being or one's ability to handle the challenge. This book was written to share humble reflections on some of my experiences as a caregiver for my mother, Grace. Caregiving is not something that I planned to do; however, I did feel that I would be "the one" to care for Mom should the need arise. As may be the case with others, caregiving for a parent is a learning and growing process. Sure, I took care of my son, but this level of care is truly not the same. In this instance, this is the person who cared for me, and now the roles are reversed. Therefore, I wish to share some of my experiences with hopes that others will embrace the honor of caregiving and realize that they are not alone. Simply put, it is rewarding and worth every effort, for I have come to accept that caregiving is an act of love and service, which is a powerful combination.

This book is not intended to diagnose, cure, solve, or save anyone from specific concerns which may occur. However, it is my intent to share a few experiences that may provide encouragement for moving gracefully through time, with purpose and intent, while caring for a loved one.

At the end of most chapters, a section entitled **"Graceful Care"** is there to offer suggestions or strategies to try or consider, which are noted as follows:

Carefully consider…

Avoid perhaps…

Reflect on your feelings…

Enrich your experience…

"**C**arefully consider" suggests something for the caregiver to contemplate, to ponder, or to which they can give some thought. "**A**void perhaps" are my mishaps, missteps, mistakes, or mis-thoughts, which can happen from time to time. "**R**eflect on your feelings" recommends that the caregiver think honestly about their internal journey, perhaps discovering and accepting that emotion is an integral part of this process. Finally, "**E**nrich your experience" is there for those who wish to reach beyond what is witnessed and to periodically

Preface

make note of some behaviors, incidents, or occurrences; write, read, record, reflect, or do whatever it takes to grow from the moment.

Following **"Graceful Care,"** I have added "**S**criptures **to P**onder," a section that suggests supportive biblical readings that can be referenced for encouragement. Meditating on God's Word can offer a deeper understanding of the content and inspire further study. This book does not provide clinical diagnoses or all-inclusive remedies to any medical concerns; it does, however, offer sincere reflections from my heart.

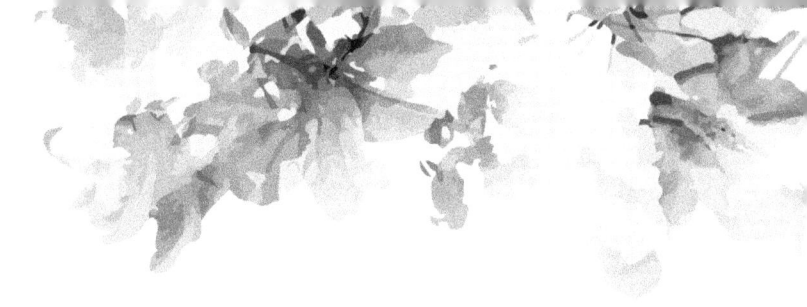

CHAPTER 1
Growing Up with Grace

Growing up with Grace, my mother, encapsulates a world of education, church, the arts, and strict discipline; our job was to do well in school. We attended elementary school, where our father was the dietician. He had mastered the art of cooking and utilized his talents as a chef and caterer. We also attended the Baptist church near our home. Mom ruled our upbringing with a stern look, her left hand, and a hairbrush, nicely packaged in love, commitment, and perseverance. That is right, no belt, no strap, no stick, or paddle—a hairbrush! Additionally, there were piano and dance lessons during the week or on weekends, and a Saturday reading club, as required by my mother.

As I recall, I was the child in the neighborhood and the sibling in my family who always wanted to play school, inspired by my mother. When I found it difficult to elicit my playmates as students, my dolls were a great substitute (perhaps the best kind because they did not talk back). My dolls also served another especially important role in my life. My best friend and I loved to play with dolls, and a part of that play included designing and sewing doll clothes with the fabric remnants from our mothers' sewing. This is something that I acquired from my mother. When she was not out shopping for finery for her children, she was at home making clothes for us, sometimes by recycling items from her personal wardrobe. This skill eventually led me to make some of my clothes as early as elementary school, using a hand needle and thread. By sixth grade, I had graduated to my mother's black electric Singer sewing machine. I was thrilled that she entrusted me with this piece of machinery. I did not know at the time that I would later use my skill as a "seamstress" to design and make costumes for my fellow dancers and dance students.

Education is important in our family. My mother inspired me to teach. The inspiration grew from observing my mother's dedication, passion, and commitment to excellence in teaching. My mother, a retired Spanish, and Social Studies teacher, was among the first in our family to graduate from college. My mother raised seven children, six of whom graduated from college. My siblings and I were in school, even at home. So, my playtime

often involved "playing school" or reading a favorite book.

To encourage our artistic development, Mom enrolled the girls in piano classes. My sisters exhibited talent for piano, while I struggled halfway through the *Teaching Little Fingers to Play* (John Thompson's Modern Course for the Piano) music book. Eventually, I quit! You see, my *little fingers* were tired of getting popped every time I missed a note! The fact that Mom did not believe in idle minds, and that I was not displaying any proficiency for the piano, meant I had to find something that I could do. When students from the local college came to the community recreation center to offer dance classes, this marked the beginning of a new chapter in my life. My sisters seemed to have a natural knack for dance; I really had to work at it, but I did not mind. Dance for me presented a desirable challenge.

During the middle grades, I decided to join the band and play an instrument from the woodwind family, the clarinet. This experience required much practice and commitment. I played well enough to hold *first chair* (lead clarinet for the section) for a brief period and learned to read music (a little). However, that was short lived once I became a cheerleader in ninth grade; at that point, my life revolved around ball games.

During my tenth-grade year, my family moved to central Florida. Eventually, a new boy's club was built in our subdivision, but the girls were not invited to attend. Fortunately, the director's wife, a dance and drama major and graduate of Spelman College, held classes at the club twice a week for the boys *and girls*. She would train the neighborhood children who expressed an interest in dance and drama. Then, when she thought we were ready, she would have us perform for someone, somewhere, including civic organizations and local events.

After a while, we outgrew the boy's club; we moved to a new location and started a neighborhood performing arts school, where the teens and young adults were soon gainfully employed. We continued to study the arts, worked for the school during the summer, and performed throughout the southern states. Time away from home was an unassailable reflection of my growing passion for the arts. My mother was truly an arts advocate; however, the increasing demand on my time caused her concern. Eventually, she decided to investigate my time-consuming activities, and before long, she had become a new cast member! My mother's investigation revealed a group of hard workers who were passionate about the arts. She allowed me to continue working with the program, and the experiences afforded me were priceless.

By the time I reached high school, I knew for sure that my desire was to teach. I could go

to school during the day and dance and act in the evening. Upon entering college, after expressing my desire to teach, I was determined to become the best teacher I could be, and to teach my students to do their best and follow their dreams.

During my internship as a teacher, I recall my "first" arts-integrated activity, with a group of first graders when they were learning to count by fives. When the supervising teacher stepped out of the room, I proceeded to add movement to help teach the five multiples, and when the teacher returned, she was thrilled to hear the students' successful counting recitation. I do not recall whether we repeated the activity; however, the first graders were pleased with themselves and happy to see the positive response from their teacher. That was the fall of 1977, and I have been a believer in the powerful impact of incorporating the arts ever since.

In 1979, I accepted a position as teacher of the gifted, and the arts made its way into my curriculum through creative activities and stage productions. Before leaving that position in 1986, I had auditioned for a professional dance company in Atlanta (the director was also a Spelman graduate). Between 1983 and 1991, I performed as a dancer with the company, while working for a tutoring franchise. During my tenure with the dance company, we traveled to schools, teaching children about the culture of Africa through dance, music, and narrative, for a program that provided arts events to schools and the community.

My belief in the arts and the experiences that I had as a child were instilled in me by my mother. Although limited, at the age of eighty-nine, Mom would still break out in song and speak with much expression. I observed my mom as a teacher, as I made doll clothes during child's play, danced at every opportunity, and made an occasional stage appearance in a few local dramatic presentations. It seems my destiny was set; the arts were ingrained in my heart, soul, and spirit.

I can tell you that Mom ensured that my siblings and I experienced the arts somewhere in our lives. What I did not know was that I would eventually experience the art of caring for someone who had cared for me. And quite frankly, I had to engage some of what I have learned to care for my mother, Ms. Grace, and for that I am profoundly grateful. As you read the reflections in this book, please remember that I am simply sharing my experiences and claim no medical expertise; I am just my mom's baby girl, Donna Olivia!

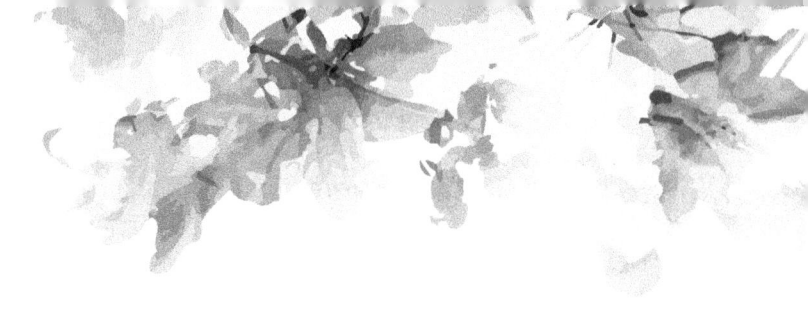

CHAPTER 2
Mom Lives with Me Now

The first time that Mom came to live with me, she came willingly; it was like one of her many travels, a quick trip, or a much-needed vacation. For example, when Mom traveled to Mexico, she returned with a wealth of knowledge, and she was more than interested in sharing what she had learned. When Mom traveled from state to state, she would take pictures, make slides, and share her experience with family and students; I guess that was the social studies teacher in her. Slides during those days were transparent images that were placed in a special carousel and projected on a screen for viewing. She absolutely loved sharing her knowledge with others.

One day while rummaging through my things, I came across a postcard from Mom, one that I had totally forgotten. During her travels, she had visited Southfork. Yes, *the* Southfork, you know, JR's Southfork (OK, maybe it was somewhere similar, but I still was excited), and she had taken a moment to send me that card. Does anyone even do that anymore? It was so cool to get a postcard in the mail. It basically said that she had visited Southfork and saw JR's room; what a precious keepsake. The point is, she loved traveling and sharing her experiences.

Once Mom had settled in with me at my home, we both needed to readjust. Ms. Grace knew that she was not at home and was probably not going back anytime soon; I, on the other hand, had to accept that she was not particularly excited about it. So, not being the neatest or most organized person, I adjusted a few things downstairs, purchased a bed, and attempted to make Mom as comfortable as possible. However, that was not the challenge—cooking was! I was trying to satisfy Mom's appetite and taste palette. Although she was not hard to please, let me just say that where my culinary skills were concerned, some days were better than others.

When Mom visited once before, we were able to go to church, eat out occasionally, go shopping, and visit the school where I worked to watch the students perform; she was simply a social butterfly. She would talk with those who would listen, with some folks finding her to be quite entertaining. On occasion, we would dress alike, and be proud to sport our "twin" look. Mom even enjoyed speaking

Spanish from time to time with her new acquaintances. However, things would soon change, and we both had to adjust to our new way of living.

Mom and I basically live downstairs in the house. She went from walking around in her own home with assistance to becoming immobile around mine, from dressing herself to being dressed, and from feeding herself to being fed via peg tube. The changes that Mom experienced really took a mental and spiritual, as well as physical, adjustment for me to learn to care for her. I had always thought I was a patient person, certainly imperfect, but patient. Now, I had a true opportunity to test my fortitude.

The changes that Mom experienced really took a mental and spiritual, as well as physical, adjustment for me to learn to care for her.

Graceful Care:

Carefully consider...taking time to reflect on precious moments; it can be very uplifting.

Avoid perhaps...immediately purging the personal belongings. Some things are worth keeping. You just may find it has sentimental value when you least expect it.

Reflect on your feelings…How would you feel if someone got their hands on your things and simply started tossing them with little or no regards for its value to you? We understand that some things may have to go, but not everything!

Enrich your experience…by journaling the precious moments that you want to remember.

Scriptures **to P**onder

Matthew 10:11-12 2 Corinthians 5:1

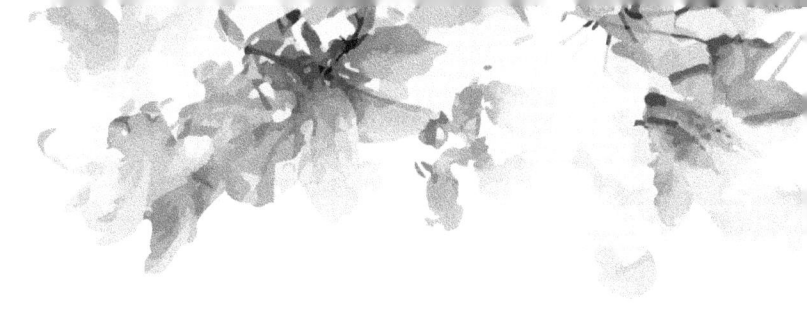

CHAPTER 3
Feeding Time

Feeding Mom was a challenge for me; you see, I was not a great cook—I am not even close! But that did not stop me from trying. Sometimes I resorted to "quick meals" because she seemed to like the taste. I would add vegetables, trying to balance her meals. Mom liked apple juice, so I kept that on hand as well. That worked for a while, and honestly, I did not expect that to change, but it did.

While Mom was able to sit up and eat, she took pride in feeding herself. The hospice service had provided a table for her, and she had moved from fork to spoon; this helped to secure the food better as she lifted it from the plate or bowl. I did not expect that her eating with a fork would change, but it did.

As I observed her struggling to get the spoon to her mouth, I thought of a way to modify the table to assist with her feeding. Off to the local home improvement store I went, and I snooped around until I found the supplies that I thought I would need to complete the project. I secured a small board, approximately 14"x20", and a couple of large clamps and created an extension for the table. This worked out quite well, at least until Mom could no longer sit up. I did not expect that her ability to sit up would end, but it surely did.

Once Mom became bedridden, she had to be fed. Aside from the fact that I was not a good cook, feeding time was fine. That is, at least until she refused to eat. Then I had to be creative in feeding her, to insure she was eating and taking her medicine. For example, Mom often had applesauce with her oatmeal for breakfast, and a taste of vanilla ice cream to take her medicine after dinner. I would have to crush her pills, sprinkle it in the applesauce or ice cream, and serve it to Mom spoon by spoon. That worked for a while until she refused to eat. I did not ever foresee her refusing to eat; I simply did not expect that to happen, but it did.

Once Mom was placed on a feeding tube, her weight and nutrition stabilized. I cannot say whether she missed eating or not. That, I just do not know. But I do know that she was more vibrant, energetic, and strong, perhaps due to the daily feedings of her nutritional cocktail. From time to time, I had to remind myself that she may not understand or recall what was going on with the feeding tube.

Feeding Time

Sometimes when I am feeding her, she needs reassurance that I am not trying to hurt her or put something in her eyes; I have assured Mom that I mean her no harm and remind her that I am there to help.

Over time, I became a **novice expert** (if there is such a thing) on some aspects of caregiving. Changing and administering meds, wound care, feeding, and looking out for infamous bedsores were among my major learning curves. I am still struggling with and working on making the bed with Mom still in it; that has been difficult for me. However, God is seeing me through it all, every step of the way! I am convinced that I would not have made it through this process without Him! Think about it—taking care of Mama. Not your child, your mother. Somehow, it is a good thing and a God thing!

> *I am convinced that I would not have made it through this process without Him! Think about it—taking care of Mama. Not your child, your mother. Somehow, it is a good thing and a God thing!*

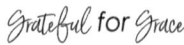

Graceful Care:

Carefully consider…modifying something that is not working; adjust as needed.

Avoid perhaps…criticizing yourself about the things you did not foresee, regardless of whether you are a novice or an experienced caregiver.

Reflect on your feelings…think about someone standing over you with a foreign object in hand and you are not familiar with the process. Wouldn't you ask a few questions? Probably.

Enrich your experience…Look for creative ways to comfort your loved one.

Scriptures **to P**onder

Philippians 4:6-7 2 Timothy 1:7

CHAPTER 4

Brushing Mom's Hair

Mom loves to have her hair brushed; it is a special treat. She no longer sees the hairdresser, who conveniently lived about ten minutes from her home. Since she was unable to style her cotton-soft hair as she wished, the Certified Nursing Assistant (CNA) would do a weekly, no-rinse cleansing, followed by a good brushing, which Mom really seemed to enjoy. Sometimes she would flinch when you came near her face or eyes, but once she felt that brush stroke, she would say, "That feels so good." Occasionally, I would put those pink-and-black sponge rollers in her hair, the ones that she once used, and the result would be beautiful, silver curls.

One day, a substitute for Mom's CNA came to work with her; I was not at home when she got there, but I arrived before she left. When I walked downstairs, together the sub and the sitter were washing Mom's hair using a bed tub, shampoo, pouring cup, and towel. Even though this was difficult to do on a regular basis, it was a welcomed change. Just think about it—when someone washes your hair or scratches your scalp, how does it feel to you? What I had to remember was that there were some things that she may still enjoy, and I was not necessarily going to know until I tried them. So, gentle massages to the scalp or gently stroking her forehead or holding her hand and singing, even with my voice, could be soothing. Just having someone work on your hair simply feels good, and it did to her as well. Whenever she had a chance, she would scratch her scalp (just as any of us might do); however, I had to monitor that. The point here is that I had to learn to be observant; this was critical in the process of caregiving, and it really took growth on my part.

Graceful Care:

Carefully consider... finding ways to comfort your loved one; although the hair

The point here is that I had to learn to be observant; this was critical in the process of caregiving, and it really took growth on my part.

may be shedding, stimulation of the scalp feels good.

Avoid perhaps…brushes with hard bristles because the scalp may be extra sensitive; a soft brush can work just as well.

Reflect on your feelings…If you have you ever had someone brush your hair or scratch your scalp, you know how that feels. It is pampering that can go a long way.

Enrich your experience…by observing the reaction to the "pampering" of choice. Perhaps now, two folks are feeling exceptionally well, the giver and the receiver.

Scriptures **to P**onder

Psalm 71:21 2 Corinthians 1:3-4

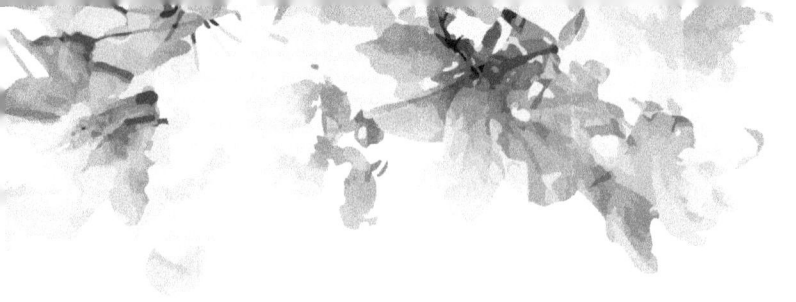

CHAPTER 5
Hats, Lots and Lots of Hats!

Mom did not mind having her hair done, but she loved her hats! When Mom came to live with me, she had a few basic items with her to make her feel comfortable, and among those items were her hats! Mom loved to wear hats. Whether it was for church, a ballgame, or any other occasion, she sported her hats and caps.

I collected coffee mugs, and Mom collected hats. When we went to church, I made sure she was wearing a matching hat. Mom was "foxy," and it made me happy to see her dressed, which is something she did quite well until she could not do it on her own. Sometimes we would coordinate the way we were dressed, except she would have on a hat! I do not know if she was raised that way or if it was simply her special attribute.

Mom had hats for church, hats for special occasions, caps for sporting events, and both

for daily wear, some of which were souvenirs from her travels; you name it, and she seemed to have a hat or cap for it. It was not that she wanted to cover her hair, which was silver and soft like cotton candy. No, she was simply being Mrs. Grace.

As a schoolteacher, Mom was very particular about how she dressed. Consequently, she had clothes galore. Sometimes I wondered if she ever wore the same thing twice. Seriously, Dad (my stepfather who was a master carpenter, builder, and craftsman at the time) designed and built a special walk-in closet for her clothes and shoes. Then I realized what her secret was... she shopped for sales, and now, I find myself doing the same. I am so grateful for this lesson. Maybe I learned this one a bit too well!

Some folks like shoes and some folks, like my mother, love hats! One night, she asked for a hat, and I gave her one to wear—a beige knit hat. I put it on her head, and she thanked

> *Mom was "foxy," and it made me happy to see her dressed, which is something she did quite well until she could not do it on her own.*

me. Eventually, she took it off and placed it in front of her on the bed. Later, when it was time for me to adjust her in the bed, she appeared to be sleeping. I removed the hat from the bed so that it would not get lost in the covers. When I got ready to move her (April 5, 2018, at 1:45 a.m.), she opened her eyes and said, "Where is my hat?" I was so shocked! I was surprised that she remembered, because one of her struggles has been with short-term memory. Yes, I was surprised, but more than that, I was proud of her. In my opinion, that was her short-term memory kicking in! Some may say that it was simply a coincidence. Hum…maybe, but I would rather think that her mind was in that special place at that time. It was a beautiful moment.

Graceful Care:

Carefully consider…that even though your loved one was bedbound, that did not mean that they did not still want their special things. What harm could that possibly be for what appeared to bring joy? So, select a few of your loved one's favorite hats (or another favorite item) and make it a conversation piece. The responses may surprise you.

Avoid perhaps…moving all items (that are not harmful) out of their presence. That is not too much to ask.

Hats, Lots And Lots Of Hats!

Reflect on your feelings...How would you feel having some of your favorite things around while you are convalescing or seeking respite? Think about the joy and comfort it may bring.

Enrich your experience...when you select that special item/hat, try locating a picture of him/her with or wearing that item, then start a conversation.

Scriptures **to P**onder

Psalm 16:1 20:4-5

CHAPTER 6
Mom's Wise Words (Grace-isms)

Mom has special words of wisdom, and it is just like her to share the wisdom with those who are willing to listen. I cannot say enough how grateful I am for my mother. Ms. Gracie, as she is fondly called by some, had her special ways about herself, and that includes her special sayings. For example, she often said, "To thine own self be true" (from Shakespeare's *Hamlet*), or "Ain't nothing wrong with doing right." Sometimes there were unexpected remarks like, "You're always talking, but you have something to say." One day, Mom blurted out, "You don't need a lot of people; you just need your true self." Now, whether these are self-created or borrowed, the words certainly have implications for life lessons. Mom's words of wisdom were intended to instruct, guide, or help us build confidence in ourselves; her "Grace-isms" were incredibly special and meaningful.

Mom's Wise Words (grace-isms)

Interestingly, even in her Alzheimer's stage of life, she did not hesitate to impart some words of wisdom. Sometimes she seemed to create these words of wisdom to fit the situation. Mom seemed to use words of encouragement as a motivator for others. She encouraged me during my postgraduate work by telling me not to let anything hold me back. There, my mother of eighty-eight years said to me words that would prove to be pivotal to my doctoral journey. How grateful I was that God would use her like that. From time to time, doubt would creep into my thoughts, but I was glad to know that she was still there urging me on to the finish line!

> *Mom's words of wisdom were intended to instruct, guide, or help us build confidence in ourselves; her "Grace-isms" were incredibly special and meaningful.*

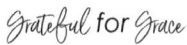

Graceful Care:

C*arefully consider…*Embrace and cherish the encouraging words that you may hear from your loved one.

A*void perhaps…*feeling sad because you recall the wisdom she imparted; instead, rejoice in how the wisdom may have guided your life.

R*eflect on your feelings…*Think about how the specially imparted words affected you, whether they made you laugh, cry, or simply be happy that your ears were the recipient. Search for joy or gratitude somewhere in the midst.

E*nrich your experience…*Write those words as often as you can and reflect on them; you will never know when they may come in handy.

Scriptures **to P**onder

Job 12:12 Proverbs 16:16; 31:26
1 Corinthians 12:8

CHAPTER 7
Struggling with Memory

When Mom forgets who I am, I smile and say something like "Yes, I am your daughter, your baby girl." Then she will look at me in amazement and be so pleased to know that I am her daughter. Sometimes, she would ask me who my mother is, and I would answer her by saying, "Grace, you are." Then the biggest smile would come across her face as she would digest, for the moment, what I had just said to her. Admittedly, this is an extremely difficult aspect of her illness. It is difficult because sometimes I am in denial; I do not want to face the reality that my mother does not recognize me. Nevertheless, I had to accept it to move forward with her care. I continued to hope, however, that somehow, I would be able to change this stage of her life, or that maybe research would soon discover a cure or some brilliant means of reversing the disease.

Mom's Alzheimer's went from somewhat remembering who I was to not knowing at all, and from asking who I was to not asking me at all. My responses sometimes brought tears to her eyes; I restrained mine. This was painful to watch and witness. I wanted to pick up the phone to reach out to someone so that they could reassure *me* that I had done nothing wrong. But there was no such luck, at least not for the moment. I had to deal with her reaction to the response I had given her, then figure out a different way to handle her question the next time.

Although the memory is waning, Mom does not seem as concerned about it now. As a matter of fact, she seems quite content with where she is mentally (if that is even possible). For instance, she would awaken on some mornings speaking to someone, singing

> *Mom's Alzheimer's went from somewhat remembering who I was to not knowing at all, and from asking who I was to not asking me at all. My responses sometimes brought tears to her eyes; I restrained mine.*

a song, and maybe even suggesting that she needed to get up (and go somewhere). Sometimes she would say, "Did someone say, 'Grace'?" because she thought that she had heard her name called. That certainly put me in a quandary because she still knew her name.

There are fewer questions now from Mom, but she will tell you how she is feeling through words, moans, or her priceless expressions. However, some things seem ingrained in her spirit. She may struggle with memory; nonetheless, she will let you know where NOT to touch her! One morning, the nurse was checking Mom's vitals and needed to listen to her heartbeat. She came near Mom's chest area, and in that Ms. Grace tone, she said to the nurse, "Don't do that." The nurse was so tickled that she had to stop for a moment just to laugh. Fortunately, she was quite familiar with the prudish side of Mom and therefore had to back off, if only for a moment. So, if we were keeping score between Mom and Alzheimer's disease, that would, without question, be a point for Ms. Grace!

Graceful Care:

Carefully consider…not looking too disappointed in your loved one's presence when you see them struggling with memory.

Grateful for Grace

Avoid perhaps…getting sad, upset, or disappointed that they cannot recall who you are. Meditate on the time when they did know.

Reflect on your feelings…How do you feel when someone makes you feel bad? Consider this before you react in their presence; they generally mean no harm.

Enrich your experience…Be creative with getting their mind off what they do not remember and focus on what they can remember, or something pleasant for the current moment.

Scriptures **to P**onder

James 1:12 Galatians 6:9 Romans 5:3-5

CHAPTER 8
The Blessed Decision

As a caregiver, I sometimes had to make tough decisions. Deciding how to keep Mom nourished was one of them, and when Mom started rejecting her food, this meant that getting her meds was going to be difficult as well. She would tighten her lips and shake her head to let me know that she was not interested in eating. I had tried several strategies to get her to eat—applesauce in oatmeal, even meds in vanilla ice cream, all while trying to monitor her sugar intake. All of this stopped working, and she stopped talking.

The day after Thanksgiving 2017, Mom would not eat, and by Saturday, I decided that she needed to go to the hospital. By the time the paramedics arrived to transport her, I was distraught. Fortunately, my niece agreed to meet me at the hospital. Mom was listless, and I had calmed down enough to explain why she needed to be there. To complicate matters, Mom not only was not eating but also had a bedsore that we had been nursing. I felt that she was slowly fading away.

The doctor explained that he would need to poke and prod to ascertain the problem; we asked him to do all that they could to help her. It was not long before Mom was talking to the medical team and telling them what *not* to do to her (Remember, when she arrived, she was not talking at all). Several days later, we were discussing a "peg tube" for her. Once the medical team justified their recommendation, the family decided that it was best for her. After twelve days and $72,000 later, they were ready to send Mom home from the hospital. However, I asked that they arrange for respite care; I needed time for the professionals to train me on how to manage that feeding tube. My request was granted. I made daily visits to the hospice facility, and about eight days later, Mom came home.

I had juggled my schedule to suit the nurses so that I would be there to learn this new technique. Truthfully, I was frightened out of my wits. What if I made a mistake? What if something happened that I was not prepared to handle? What if this feeding tube thing did not work? I did not want to feel anxious about it, but I was worried.

Twenty days later, she had returned with two new procedures, a catheter, and a feeding tube, a decision that was made collectively.

The Blessed Decision

Mom seemed to adjust well to both, while I, on the other hand, struggled with concerns for what she must have been feeling. I was also so afraid of handling her wrong or hurting her with tubes coming from two places too many! I suppose it was natural to feel that way. I wrestled with this decision that we made as a family, and I finally resolved that putting Mom on a feeding tube was critical to sustaining life for her and was therefore a blessed decision! Mom rested more peacefully, and whenever my "mommy duty" was done for the moment, I looked forward to my rest; Mom appeared content and peaceful when she slept, and I aimed for the same. Sometimes it worked, sometimes it did not.

> *I wrestled with this decision that we made as a family, and I finally resolved that putting Mom on a feeding tube was critical to sustaining life for her and was therefore a blessed decision!*

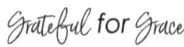

Graceful Care:

Carefully consider…a calm approach when new situations are on the rise.

Avoid perhaps…speculating on the new changes.

Reflect on your feelings…Do new procedures cause you to become anxious? Be honest about it and use the energy to address your concerns.

Enrich your experience…by consulting someone more knowledgeable than yourself and taking note of any resources suggested for future reference.

Scriptures **to P**onder.

Deuteronomy 5:16 Ephesians 6:1-4

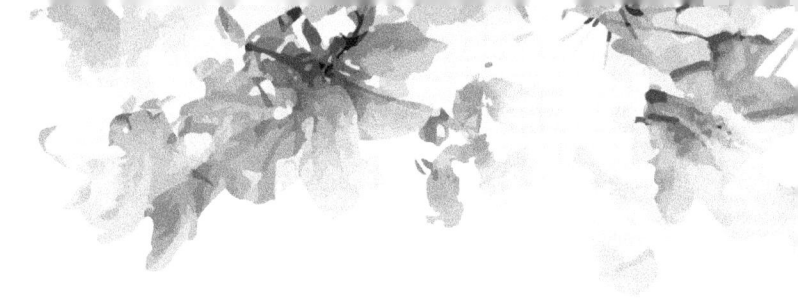

CHAPTER 9
Mom's Reflections (Teaching Still)

Mom continued to thrive because of the "blessed decision" made on her behalf. One evening, I heard her talking and noticed that she appeared to be speaking to students. In fact, she was teaching! I listened more intently as she seemed to relive some of her classroom moments. It was so vivid to her, the students, and the kids that she referenced. She would ask them to take out their books or to get a sheet of paper. One night, I even heard her encouraging a student to get up and do their best and to have confidence. I can only imagine the kind of teacher she was. I remember when she would grade papers or give me instructions for making her bulletin boards (which became one of my favorite things to do as a teacher). Late at night, I can hear her saying some of the words that she must have spoken to her students. One conversation went something like this:

> "Boys and girls, I need for each of you to take out a sheet of paper, because each of you should have your materials and be prepared for class today. You should always come to class prepared with your materials, ready to work. Go ahead and take out your books as well. Come on now, let's settle down and get busy so that we can get down to work."

Observing her as she spoke these words was utterly amazing; my mom was still teaching. My listening to her was an introspective approach to accepting this phase of her condition. Except for the fact that no one was there (at least I could not see anyone), Mom was on it; she had total control of that invisible classroom. One day, I asked to whom she was speaking, and I

my mom was still teaching. My listening to her was an introspective approach to accepting this phase of her condition.

Mom's Reflections (teaching Still)

finally realized that I was only interrupting class, and simply needed to be quiet and just listen.

Mom also has a sense of humor when she teaches. Every now and then, you may hear her imitate the students in her own way to bring about laughter or a hearty chuckle. Even though Mom was encouraging and had a funny side, I felt that it may have been difficult for me had I been in her class, as her expectations were high! I guess being in the class of "life" with her was enough of a blessing for me, and for that I am grateful.

Graceful Care:

Carefully consider…finding ways to create humor and laughter with your loved one.

Avoid perhaps…dreading the characteristics of Alzheimer's or any other disease and instead look for the lessons that you can learn from them.

Reflect on your feelings…Are there any teachers in your life who encouraged you? What lessons have you learned from a teacher that you can apply to your life today?

Enrich your experience…If there was a teacher or someone who encouraged you along the way, this may be a great time to say thank you to them or make it known to someone in their family.

Grateful for *Grace*

Scriptures **to P**onder

Proverbs 22:6 Matthew 19:14

CHAPTER 10
Getting Me through School

As previously mentioned, I was inspired to teach by my mother, who is a staunch believer in education. When I decided to pursue my "final" postgraduate degree, Mom was not living with me at the time; however, my steps were evidence that I embraced her educational influences; her belief in a good education still resonated within me. As a child, I knew that I wanted to teach and have a positive impact on students as much as possible. To do that, I needed to become a lifelong learner. That too came from my mother, who consistently had us being "enriched" year-round in some academic setting.

My son, Joseph, who often keeps late hours, also knows the importance of education. When he was busy preparing for the excitement and challenges of his high school senior year, one night, he noticed I was discouraged about my comprehensive exam. So, he took a moment to say, "Well, it's not like you are just sitting around; you are working and trying to do something productive." During the early morning hours, Joseph would come from his room and see me hard at work at the dining room table, and every now and then, he would say something. One night (or perhaps I should say morning), he walked through the dining room and saw me at the table, struggling to stay awake. He looked at me, paused, and said, "I know what you need." He then proceeded to the kitchen to make a cup of hot chocolate for me. I was so touched by his action and sensitive attitude toward the situation that it nearly brought me to tears (not to mention that hot chocolate has a way of being a cure-all). I was so thankful to my son for his encouraging words and the hot cocoa that accompanied those words during the late-night hours.

Now that Mom was living with us, my son was not the only one pushing me to the finish line. One morning while working on Chapter 1 of my dissertation, I had the privilege of having my mother, the "ultimate educator," sitting in front of me, as I was now her caregiver. At eighty-eight years of age, she looked up at me and asked, "How far advanced are you in your education?" I responded by telling her that I was working on my Ph.D. She turned around in her wheelchair, gently nodded her head, and said to me, "Well, alright. Well, my

Getting Me Through School

advice to you is to never give in and never give up, stay on the move, don't let anything hold you back." The words of my mother, who was now diagnosed with Alzheimer's disease, had provided the additional confirmation and motivation for the work I was doing. I had to look forward and move on to completion. At eighty-eight, she was *still* encouraging and *still* watching me! When I was admitted to the Ph.D. program for Curriculum and Instruction, I knew I would need special support and encouragement, and I am glad to know that I had that support in my mother and my son. Furthermore, it was good to know that my mother, in the early stage of her Alzheimer's diagnosis, still exhibited the mental capacity to express her concern for my education.

Furthermore, it was good to know that my mother, in the early stage of her Alzheimer's diagnosis, still exhibited the mental capacity to express her concern for my education.

Graceful Care:

Carefully consider… answering questions about yourself as

truthfully as possible (should your loved one ask). You never know what advice may follow.

Avoid perhaps…dodging the reality of your new and current responsibility as a caregiver; the care can be a two-way street.

Reflect on your feelings…Have you ever experienced an occasion where a loved one offered kind and encouraging words to you? This could be a great time for gratitude.

Enrich your experience…Think back on the kind and encouraging advice you have received from the person in your care; if it had a positive effect on you, pass it on!

Scriptures **to P**onder

Psalm 25:4-5; 32:8 Proverbs 3:5-6; 16: 9
Jeremiah 29:11

CHAPTER 11
A Little More Time Together

When Mom started living with me, I had to spend time trying to explain why she could not leave my house and go home. I have often reminded her of who I am. Whenever I tell her that I am "her," Donna Olivia, I may get a smile, a look of concern, or a look of sadness as if she wonders why she did not remember that on her own. Generally, I would embrace the sincerity of the moment and move on, but on one occasion, I had a reversed situation, which gave me something different to consider. On October 21, 2019, Mom called my name. Although I cannot explain why, it certainly got my attention. I rushed to her side and took a good look at her to see if I was dreaming or hearing things. And for just a moment, there was fleeting hope. Mom had spent many years developing the minds of students and even channeling their minds to think positively about themselves.

And now, she was struggling with her own mental state. Yet for me, this situation presented hope that maybe her memory would return.

I did not want to alarm or frighten her, but I felt a need to say, "Thank you, Mom. Thank you for recognizing that I am here, and for calling my name." When we were young, Mom would call for one of us by calling all the girls' names. She would say, "Cheryl… uh, uh, Pammy…uh, uh, I mean Donna," with the cutest little stutter. But rest assured, she would get the right one eventually. It meant so much to me to hear her say, "Donna." It was as if she had just given us *a little more time together*.

It meant so much to me to hear her say, "Donna." It was as if she had just given us a little more time together.

Graceful Care:

Carefully consider…being in the moment, and letting it flow.

A Little More Time Together

Avoid perhaps…stopping to correct or showing confusion on your face when you hear something unexpected.

Reflect on your feelings…How do pleasantries make you feel? Then help your loved one get as many pleasantries as possible.

Enrich your experience…You may want to write these special moments down, then reflect on them when you want something to smile about.

Scriptures **to P**onder

Proverbs 17:6 Ephesians 4:2-3

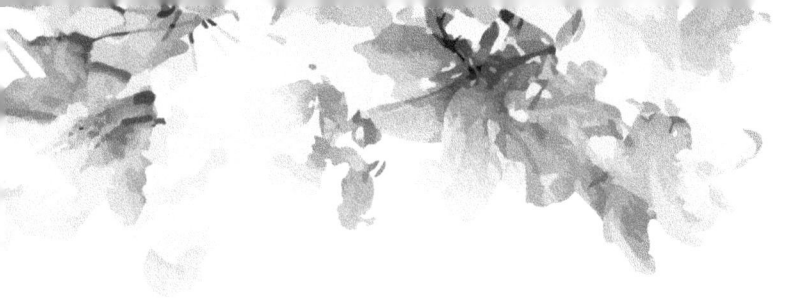

CHAPTER 12
Taking Mom Out

Mom has her way of showing that she is still in the present moment, for she had yet another surprise waiting for me. One night while waiting to pick up my son from one of his activities, Mom and I stopped by a local cantina for a short outing. Mom used a cane then and was quite mobile. I was somewhat nervous about this stop; however, that soon changed. You see, Mom was always on the go, so she was no stranger to being out. You might even say she was a social butterfly. Outside of church and school (work), she worked with an organization called the Agricultural Labor Program International (ALPI) and did so for over thirty years.

Mom did not mind socializing. As a matter of fact, I remember going out with her during one of my trips back home. Imagine that, hanging out with Mom. It was always in good taste though; after all, she was Ms. Grace.

Taking Mom Out

Anyway, we pulled up to the door of the cantina. We got out of the car, and as we approached the door, you could hear the music, compliments of the DJ. I could tell that she liked the atmosphere (Spanish teacher, cantina…get it?). Some of the patrons politely greeted her as she enjoyed walking through the door. We were only planning to be there a short while, so as soon as my son called, we prepared to leave. As Mom stood up, a song came on that she could not resist. Although we were leaving, she just had to dance a step or two. Mom started strutting to the beat, toward the door, and the crowd went wild! With her cane in one hand and her purse in the other, she

Mom did not mind socializing. As a matter of fact, I remember going out with her during one of my trips back home. Imagine that, hanging out with Mom. It was always in good taste though; after all, she was Ms. Grace.

singlehandedly stole the hearts of the cantina patrons that night. She would dance, then pause, dance, and pause again until she reached the door. Some people cheered her on, while others used their cell phones to record the moment. Then she added one of her "Grace-isms," stating, "To keep on moving, you have to keep on grooving." Just as she was about to exit, one of the managers came over and acknowledged her exuberant presence and performance. Before she left, he declared Mom an honorary visitor of the cantina, stating that she was welcome at any time, and that whatever she ordered would be on the house. What a blast it was to see Ms. Grace, once again, "cut a step!"

Graceful Care:

Carefully consider…taking your loved one out if he/she is mobile and able. I have noted people stopping to watch us together or as we walk across the parking lot. I truly have an appreciation for those who are sensitive to our seniors and their special situation.

Avoid perhaps…feeling badly because you cannot "go" or do something because your loved one cannot go with you; think about where the real joy is and find peace there.

Reflect on your feelings…Dig deep, if necessary, to find the compassion for any situation that comes your way. It is there; it is there!

Taking Mom Out

Enrich your experience...by cuddling up with a photo album or something that brings fond memories (if applicable). Perhaps you will forget all about where you wanted to go.

Scriptures **to P**onder

Proverbs 17:22 Ecclesiastes 3:4; 8:15

CHAPTER 13

Never Say Never

I did not think that things would get to the point where I would need to be Mom's caregiver, but what an experience it has been thus far. There have been good days and rough days, with much uncertainty, and collectively, all are a part of the blessing of caring for a loved one. Initially, I could not fathom doing for my mother the things that she once did for me—feeding, bathing, clothing, and simply being there for me. Even in my adulthood,

There have been good days and rough days, with much uncertainty, and collectively, all are a part of the blessing of caring for a loved one.

I needed my mother to be there for me! Nevertheless, it was important for me to do all that I could to help her.

Mom is occasionally uncertain about me as her caregiver, but she would eventually calm down and allow me to care for her. For example, dressing her could be quite a task, especially when she felt that it was absolutely unnecessary for me to do so. Sometimes she would cooperate, and sometimes she would not. But just how does caring for a parent or loved one happen? Is it planned, are you nominated, or do you simply volunteer? Whatever the case, if it has ever occurred to you that you may become a caregiver, just the thought of it can be overwhelming. One may even decide that handling such a feat would be next to impossible, because the details of such circumstances can be very unpredictable. You can speculate, read about it, or even

You can speculate, read about it, or even consult with someone, but you simply do not really know how you would handle caregiving until you are in it.

consult with someone, but you simply do not really know how you would handle caregiving until you are in it.

If you have given it some thought, and you have decided that you could "never" do any caregiving, surely it is not due to the lack of love for the person; instead, caregiving simply may not be what you are cut out to do. If you know ahead of time, you may try to plan for it. Now, that may be possible, but when you are not prepared, that is quite different. If you live in close proximity to the person, you may start with dropping by to check on them, doing maintenance chores, or shopping for necessities. These things are commendable; however, they should not be compared with twenty-four-hour care.

You can see that there is much to ponder here. So, if you thought that you would "never" be able to offer continuous care for a loved one, remember <u>never</u> may reflect your confidence level for handling the challenge. If you or your family are faced with such a decision, try to follow your heart, and **never say never.** You may be surprised by the strength and courage that can come upon you with divine intervention.

Graceful Care:

Carefully consider…your decision to care for your loved one and what it may mean for you and your current lifestyle. Prayer is key.

Avoid perhaps…the "yes, you should" and "no, you shouldn't" comments. Instead, let God guide the decision.

Reflect on your feelings…What if you needed help and no one stepped up to assist you? I think no one wants to imagine that!

Enrich your experience…How do you agree to do something when you do not know what you are saying yes to? Try letting the love of God in your heart take the lead, and it can do wonders for the experience that you may encounter.

Scriptures **to P**onder

Psalm 121:1 James 1:6

CHAPTER 14

I Wondered, I Waited (and Tried Not to Worry)

I learned early on that it was not wise to guess what may or may not ever happen. I would therefore wonder and wait to see what the next day would bring. When Mom awakened in the morning, sometimes she greeted me with a smile. On those days, my objective was to keep that smile on her face. At times, that was difficult to do, considering the aches and pains that she may encounter and endure throughout the day. However, that did not deter my efforts to make her comfortable. I wondered how much my efforts would help, then waited to see the results. When my attempts were unsuccessful, I felt like a failure and that I had disappointed her. When I was able to comfort her, for the moment there was peace.

I Wondered, I Waited (and Tried Not To Worry)

On occasion, it was necessary to send Mom to respite care. Sending your son or daughter to school with a note is one thing but imagine sending a note with your mother when she goes to respite. But when your loved one is unable to verbalize their needs, a note is necessary! The time away from me was difficult. I wondered if she would miss me, and I anxiously waited for her return. Now, please understand, I had to adjust to her respite visits. The social worker helped me understand how important the "breaks" were. When Mom left the first time, one of the drivers of the medical vehicle asked how long she would be gone, and when I said, "One day," he immediately alluded to the fact that I must be new. Nonetheless, I cried as they drove away, and I prayed for understanding. I wondered if she would really be alright without me, and I waited to hear any news from the respite center.

When the decision was made to feed Mom via gastro-tube, I gave thought to several unknown circumstances. I wondered, for example, if she knew that she was not eating by mouth, and I waited for her to ask for food, but she did not. Every now and then, she would reach for the tube. Bless her heart, perhaps she was relieved that she no longer had to eat my cooking!

I also often wondered if Mom would call my name, and I waited to hear it as time ticked during the day. To her, I was Donna or Donna Olivia. I wondered and I waited. Sometimes she did call for me, but most of the time she did not. Thus, I tried not to look for it, but I knew that I would welcome the surprise when and if she did.

I eventually adjusted to the visitations from the hospice service, nurse, CNA, social worker, chaplain, and recertification nurse. There were times when I wondered when they would come, waited for them to arrive, then wondered again what I might learn during the visit. This was particularly important to me. I approached the visits with expectancy. I had my reservations about what I would learn, but I knew that I was in a different kind of school and that the wondering and waiting was a part of the process. Caring for Mom required love, patience, and "on the job" training. It was

> *Caring for Mom required love, patience, and "on the job" training. It was imperative that I learned my lessons quickly and that I learned them well.*

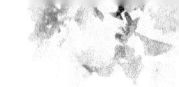

imperative that I learned my lessons quickly and that I learned them well. This was my caregiving journey, and I had to be prepared for the road trip.

Graceful Care:

Carefully consider…Although you may wonder and wait, meditate on the positive to extinguish negativity.

Avoid perhaps…trying to predict the next day or the future; instead, enjoy the present moments that you have.

Reflect on your feelings…Does wondering and waiting make you anxious? If so, rethink the time you spend with those thoughts and try replacing them with something more pleasant and less stressful.

Enrich your experience…Try preparing questions for the healthcare visitations that you may have. This can allow you as the caregiver to guide a portion of the visit.

Scriptures **to P**onder

Isaiah 40:31; 41:10 Psalm 27:14

CHAPTER 15
The New Normal

Even when wondering and waiting helps you adjust to a caregiving routine, there always seems to be new processes to learn. You see, just when I thought I had a handle on most of Mom's concerns, a pandemic changed my learning curve. Now, what do I do? Here was my now ninety-one-year-old mother, my twenty-year-old son, and two sixty-three-year-olds (my husband and I), all looking to cohabitate safely in one household. Yikes! Well,

> *You see, just when I thought I had a handle on most of Mom's concerns, a pandemic changed my learning curve.*

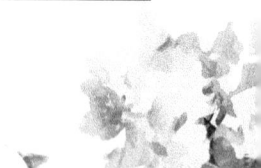

although we were not the neatest quartet, cleaning was imperative, and some guidelines had to be set. For example, wash hands often, wear masks, stand six feet apart, and use hand sanitizer. Not knowing how long the pandemic would last, such guidelines and restrictions, along with our semi-quarantined living arrangements, were now our "new normal."

As we worked to maintain our living arrangements, the hospice service, in the meantime, began to cut visits (to protect all concerned). Social workers, chaplains, and nurses were instructed to handle their visits by phone or virtually; I am sure Mom missed her visiting team during that time. However, during the pandemic, we were also blessed with a musical therapist. Periodically, Mom and I would join in as she sang so beautifully like a canary. The CNA still made her weekly rounds, and I was grateful for that!

In addition to the visiting presence of hospice were the weekly supplies. I developed the habit of wiping down anything that came through the door, including groceries, packages, and other deliveries, and that added chore included sanitizing the supplies. This "new normal" for receiving mail and deliveries was quite tedious, and sometimes so challenging to track! It was important, though, to take precautions.

My husband, a frontline worker in the transportation field, went to work five days a week. Eventually, the time came when he needed to be tested due to exposure to the virus; we were certainly dealing with the unknown here. We awaited his results with much prayer. Fortunately, the results were negative, and we were so grateful to God! From that point, we found it necessary to continue our semi-quarantined posture within our household. We had truly little choice in the matter because each day presented us with new uncertainties.

By now, the term "new normal" was being used quite often, so exactly what did that mean for us…fewer visits, no respite or services, and supplies cut? Well, the hospice services were not abrogated, but they were modified, and I had to push harder with my daily routine for Mom. In the meantime, I felt it important to be immensely grateful and to continue to be vigilant in prayer, which is my peace, my source. And to all frontline angels of mercy sent from God, THANK YOU!

Graceful Care:

Carefully consider…taking seriously guidelines for safety during a pandemic.

Avoid perhaps…watching too much news during a time like this. Now, you must be the judge about how much you can take, but the unpleasantness surrounding

The New Normal

the circumstances can tend to affect one's countenance.

Reflect on your feelings…Search yourself to honestly determine your feelings. Are you worried about what may happen? Are you afraid of the unknown? These may be realities that you must face.

Enrich your experience…While it may be difficult to tell someone not to worry, I would suggest flipping the energy and using it to reach out to a pastor, a chaplain, or a counseling service to help redirect your focus.

Scriptures **to P**onder

Isaiah 43:18-19 Romans 12:2
Ephesians 4:22-24

CHAPTER 16

You Are Not Alone

Caring for a loved one can be daunting or overwhelming, especially if you were blessed with the situation on short notice. You have decided that you want to help; however, you know that you are NOT "qualified," and that seems to resonate with you more than the loving care itself. From time to time, you may be offered helpful advice. Perhaps a family member or friend may offer a hand or their services periodically, and of course, you would like to think that would help. But the fact is you have been given the daily, twenty-four-hour charge to care for a loved one, and sometimes you may have feelings of being alone. So, where do you turn?

One recommendation is to start with an organization or association that bears the name (or a similar one) of your loves one's illness or circumstance; in Mom's case, it was the Alzheimer's Association. Additionally, an

online search can provide helpful information. I also found that I had a few friends who were experiencing health challenges with their parents as well. So, there are resources for guidance, but chose wisely and remember that the ultimate choice rests with you. Yet, with all the help in the world, you may still feel that you are alone. However, despite the uncertainties which may arise, the more you reach out for help, the more you will find that you are **not** alone.

I have found comfort in knowing that an agency cared about Mom. I found comfort in joining a caregiver's group through the church; it really helps to have someone who is sharing a similar experience to talk with. As you move through your process, research your concerns without hesitation. This was something I had to learn quickly. For example, I went through a process of learning how to work with Mom's feeding tube, but it did not occur to me that

> *I have found comfort in knowing that an agency cared about Mom. I found comfort in joining a caregiver's group through the church*

she could remove the tube. So, when she dislodged the tube from her abdominal area, I completely lost it. I was sitting on the couch, right in front of Mom's bed, when I heard a bubble, pop sound. I looked up to be sure nothing had happened in the ceiling. Then I jumped up, ran to Mom's bedside, and I think I asked her if she was OK. And as I looked at her, seeing nothing out of the ordinary, she lifted her hand up and said, "Here you go," and she kindly handed me her tube. I gasped and spastically looked around, thinking, *What do I do now?* I was NOT trained for such a time as this.

    Finally, I called the hospice center. The lady on the phone was so calm as she asked me a series of questions. I figured she did not understand, because she really did not know what had just happened. Mom was lying there with a hole in her stomach, and I could not help her. Well, the lady on the phone did understand, and she told me to call 911 and to calm down or else I would need to be on the stretcher instead of Mom. Well, that got my attention, and this certainly was a time when I felt that I needed some personal research and advice. Before ending the phone call, the hospice representative reassured me that Mom would be alright. As I reflect on that day, I felt that God sent His angels to cover me, for I was not alone.

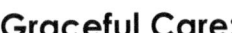

Graceful Care:

Carefully consider…calling someone when you feel alone.

Avoid perhaps…backing yourself into an "alone" corner.

Reflect on your feelings…Lonely is not a great place to be, especially when accompanied with sadness and despair. Try to push toward something more positive by expressing your need for help.

Enrich your experience…When something new enters your world of caregiving, dig a little deeper and research if possible. Remember, you are not trying to replace medical personnel; you simply want to add to your knowledge base.

Scriptures **to P**onder

Genesis 28:15 Joshua 1:9

CHAPTER 17
God's Grace

Although Mom was at the point in her life where she struggled with memory, what she did not forget was to call on God! Whether she was hurting, aching, or overwhelmingly grateful about something, she would call on God. "Oh Lord, have mercy," or "My Lord," is what she would say so sincerely. It touched my heart to know that she was still in touch and still connected to Almighty God!

Mom attended church until she absolutely could not. That is, she was unable to travel by car, and it was too dangerous to lift her. But prior to that, we would make it to service—late, but we made it there. Although she did not appear to hear every word spoken during service, she enjoyed the music and the singing. Yes, before she had to stop attending, Mom's hands clapped in church on Sunday morning!

Every now and then, Mom would break into song with generally some hymn that

God's Grace

> *Every now and then, Mom would break into song with generally some hymn that she enjoyed singing, and her favorite was "Amazing Grace."*

she enjoyed singing, and her favorite was "Amazing Grace." Mom also loved to tell the story that as a child she would go to church, and after service, her grandpa would ask what the preacher talked about. One day, she was excited to tell him the preacher talked about her because he talked about God's amazing grace. And Grandpa simply chuckled as he explained to her that it was not about her, but about God's grace. She learned a valuable lesson that day, and we are grateful that God continues to show His amazing grace to our matriarch, Ms. Grace.

Graceful Care:

Carefully consider…singing along with your loved one; they may relish the moment.

Grateful for Grace

Avoid perhaps… ignoring the singing; acknowledge it, even if it is with just a simple compliment.

Reflect on your feelings…Now, I am not asking if you can sing, but I am suggesting that you sing because whether you can or not, sometimes it is not about you. Sing with your loved one and make the best of it, or whatever it is that they enjoy.

Enrich your experience…Pay attention to the songs you may hear, then periodically lead that same song; the person in your care just may join in with you.

Scriptures **to P**onder

2 Corinthians 9:8 Hebrews 4:16 2 Peter 3:18

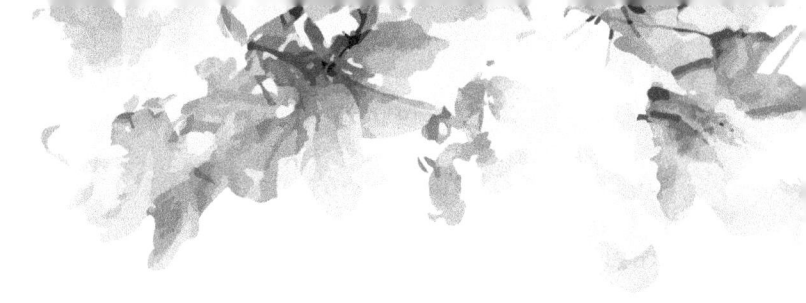

CHAPTER 18

Caring for Mom as a Work of HeART

Growing up in a household with Mama Grace included exposure to the arts. For example, we learned basic Spanish vocabulary and our multiplication tables by singing recorded songs with the specific content; the multiplication facts were rhythmic, while the Spanish content was set to a pleasant tune. We also took dance classes at the Dade Street Community Center in Tallahassee, Florida, where five of us (Cheryl, Pamela, Donna, Norbert (deceased), and Clement) were raised. My two youngest brothers (Fred Jr. and Alano), who were raised in Orlando, Florida, also had arts experiences such as drama and band.

Mom absolutely loved the arts. This is noteworthy because there were times when I found myself using the arts as a catalyst for her care. Sometimes Mom and I would sing together, or I would dance around her bed to entertain her and she would get a big kick out of that! Although she has been bedbound, I have encouraged Mom to dance with me by moving her arms or moving her head to my fictitious beat. At times when she seemed distressed, although it concerned me, I would put on the biggest "act" trying to reassure her that everything would be alright. You see, Mom was a thespian in her own right; she absolutely adored the theatrical setting. The two of us, in fact, performed in a couple of plays together. She worked hard on her roles, and I would assist. When we were in scenes together, I would make sure I knew the lines well enough, just in case she needed a little help, which rarely happened; she was masterful on stage. The point that I am making here is that whether I felt like it or not, I sometimes had to pull from my arts experiences to keep the

> *Sometimes Mom and I would sing together, or I would dance around her bed to entertain her and she would get a big kick out of that!*

caregiving atmosphere positive for Mom by staging an act.

Another challenge for me was caring for Mom's wounds. I really cared what they looked like; I was maybe even obsessive to an extent (for instance, I preferred to cut the medical tape rather than tear it), but those bandages had to be neat. As I learned wound care from the nurses who came out to visit, I tried to absorb all the fundamentals that I could. I learned why one antiseptic or cream was preferred over another. "Use this gauze," or "Let that wound breathe," the nurses would tell me. Eventually, I had to take ownership of my task at hand. I felt that the better the care, the better the results would be. Therefore, my bandages had to be neat with an aesthetic flair when possible, and with that flair came an understanding of why it needed to be applied a certain way. Visually, Mom's bandages were a work of art.

So, I danced to entertain, initiated singing (even with my voice), and put up at least a good front or act, especially at times when I was not feeling well. Hum, I wonder if that makes me a "triple threat"? Probably not, and I wish I could say that I worked my artistry every day, but that would not be true. What I can tell you, however, is that it clearly made a difference in Mom's countenance when I did, and for that I was grateful!

Graceful Care:

Carefully consider…finding the joy in this service of love that you are experiencing or embarking upon.

Avoid perhaps…letting your loved one see you bothered about any specific concern.

Reflect on your feelings…If you are feeling inadequate about the quality of care that you are offering because of what you do not know, try focusing more on the person you are helping and the good that you are doing for him/her.

Enrich your experience…Try to do something a little different each day; a little can mean a lot.

Scriptures **to P**onder

Romans 12:6-8 1 Peter 4:10

CHAPTER 19
The Little Things

Caregiving takes heart, and because you care, there is a constant urge to find strategies to aid in comforting someone. In addition to the services you may receive, you may find that there are little things, simple things that you can also do to bring comfort to someone in your care. I am mentioning this because it may be helpful to think creatively when experiencing this aspect of caregiving. What is shared here

> *In addition to the services you may receive, you may find that there are little things, simple things that you can also do to bring comfort to someone in your care.*

may not assist in your situation, but perhaps it will help spark thoughts. It may only work for one person, but the effort can mean so much to them. Here are a few examples:

BACK PILLOW

Mom's body had gotten tight and restricted, so her movements were extremely limited. This made it difficult for her to naturally turn in bed; thus, the turning had to be done with much assistance. Mom also needed extra support for her back, so I found a nice little pillow which sufficed. The hospice service offered a bed wedge, which worked as well, depending on her specific need. A little comfort can go a long way!

"BOXING" GLOVES

Mom's boxing gloves help prevent scratching. Also, since she is on a feeding tube, it keeps her from pulling it out—again. The first time she dislodged her cord, it was traumatic for me, and I was determined that it would be the last time. Now, in reality, the gloves are not those that boxers use, but that is what they looked like; they are called security or safety mitts. As a matter of fact, I once sent Mom to the respite center, with gloves and all the other things she needed to have a comfortable stay, but the gloves did not come back! I was livid, and

I tried to get them back. Unfortunately, the gloves magically disappeared, and I needed to replace them. My baby brother was visiting at the time, and when he heard me complain that Mom did not have them and why, he immediately ordered a pair; two days later, they were on my doorstep. The protective gloves were a necessity, but not everyone agreed. One day, the CNA was attempting to slide one of the gloves on Mom's hand, and she said, "Do you have to?" Moments like this remind me that Mom is still very much with us!

KNEE PILLOW

Since Mom was confined to the bed, one challenge was to keep her rotated with hopes of increasing circulation and avoiding bedsores. In addition to that, it was important to provide her with as much comfort as possible. Her knees were a big concern, so it was suggested that a pillow be placed between her knees as much as possible to relieve pressure. Interestingly, she rarely complained about her knees.

TURN

Sometimes I really hated to bother Mom when it was time to turn her, especially when she was resting, but I knew that the turning was best for her. With guidance, I needed to determine how much and how often to do the turning. Every now and then, she just slept right through whatever I was doing for her at the time. She seemed so peaceful at times like that.

MASSAGE

Take a moment to do personal research on issues that concern you. For example, as I noticed Mom's reaction to having her back rubbed or massaged, I looked for an article on how a senior might respond to a massage. The article was enlightening; seniors can enjoy pampering such as a gentle massage. So, unless it hurts, do not hesitate to investigate.

PEG TUBE GUARD

Mom's feeding tube was lodged in the center of her abdominal area, and quite frankly, it looked uncomfortable. To make the tube more comfortable when tucked away, I placed a soft sock or glove around it to avoid indentations on her skin and to keep the cold tube off her. I felt that if it were not so cumbersome, she would be less likely to bother it. A sock, a glove, the minutiae of little things do not have to be scientific to matter.

The Little Things

CELEBRATIONS

Still celebrate days that are special to the one who is in your care. Christmas, Easter, Thanksgiving, birthdays, Valentine's Day... chose one or all of them. You may also want to choose a day and declare it as <u>(name of person in your care)</u>'s day! Then do and say something special to or about them. Although this could yield an emotional response such as joy, it can also offer a break in the daily routine of caregiving. Again, the "little things" can mean so much.

Graceful Care:

Carefully consider...what you can do or what gentle touch you can add to aid in comforting your loved one.

Avoid perhaps...thinking that doing "little things" are not worthwhile.

Reflect on your feelings...Think of some of the "little things" in your life that you would hope someone would do for you.

Enrich your experience...Be creative in thinking of some "little things" for your love one; you may find joy in doing so.

Scriptures **to P**onder

1 Corinthians 13:4-7 Colossians 3:12

CHAPTER 20
Emotional Moments

In this chapter, I recommend that you tread lightly, unless of course you are resistant to tears. Not because there is something so profound or extraordinary, but that it may remind you of a similar experience or momentarily cause you to relive a precious, tender moment. The truth is, the total caregiving experience can be deemed emotional, but dwelling on that aspect of the "roller coaster ride" may not be helpful to the situation at hand. Then again, emotion just may be the catalyst that catapults you to the next moment, day, week, month, or year. Caring for someone can be likened to a roller coaster ride because there can be a variation of highs and lows, ups and downs, and every other meaningful moment that can be wedged in between. Yes, wedged, because sometimes you must remember to look for the precious moments amid trying times. Below, a few scenarios are noted.

Study with Caution. I realized early on that I had to be careful not to play doctor but instead, act as the primary observer so that I could, as accurately as possible, report any changes in Mom to the medical experts. I also needed to study, read, inquire, and conversate more to help myself get better with what I was doing. For example, I read literature, trying to understand that fine line between dementia and Alzheimer's, why bedsores develop, or understanding who Mom was talking to in the middle of the night. Reading about Mom's concerns can be both reassuring and frightening; nevertheless, it helps me to become as knowledgeable as possible, so that I can assist the medical team, not replace them.

Caring for someone can be likened to a roller coaster ride because there can be a variation of highs and lows, ups and downs, and every other meaningful moment that can be wedged in between.

Tears. One evening, Mom could not see me on the couch; truthfully, I had been napping. When I came to her bedside, she had an expression of relief. I turned away for a moment, and as I prepped to feed her, she was expressing her gratitude for my being there. When I turned back to face her, tears were in her eyes. At first, I thought I would fall apart; I wanted to cry too, but there was no time for that! I wanted to cry so badly, but I thought it would cause more concern. So, I put a big smile on my face and began to reassure her that I was there for her, that I was her daughter, and that I was there to take care of her. This changed her demeanor, and I would like to think that she felt better, if only for the moment. Seeing Mom cry was a difficult experience!

Special words. "I don't want to lose you," "I am happy you are here," "Ow, that hurts," or "It's hurting." When words like these are accompanied by a look of endearment, your heart tends to melt. During these times, I would rather not let Mom see tears in my eyes, because she still showed signs of having much compassion, and I did not want to evoke any unnecessary emotion. When you find yourself drying the tears of the person who once dried yours, it is difficult to hold your composure.

I'm frightened. Can I say that? On Wednesday nights, sometimes I felt alone. You see, there were times that my retired work

week ended on Wednesdays. After my last class, I would come home, tend to Mom, and have a little late lunch; then, after all the assistance from the hospice service was done for the day, I knew that I was all alone, and that was a frightening feeling. Well, a least that is how I felt. My son was away at school, and no one else was scheduled to come by; I did not expect any calls—just me, Mom, and the walls of the house.

If Mom was resting, then I REALLY felt alone and scared of what would happen in the next moment. So, of course, I would watch television to pass the time to get my mind off the depressing newscasts or other family matters of concern. Sometimes I would drift into deep thought, trying to think of other ways to help Mom or strategize on ways to improve on her care. I would even wonder when that surprise call would come with some family member saying that they were coming for a brief visit or even to visit for a while to sit with Mom to give me a break. Then I would be awakened from the trance by a noise from the television or the sound of Mom adjusting herself in bed. Whether you can relate to any of this or not, the truth of the matter is, you are NOT alone.

If you think about the care you have already given your loved one and did not think you could do it, or If you think about the number of times that perhaps you felt you could not go any further, you will realize that you are not alone. The lonely moments can be emotional because no one seems to be there with you, but FEAR NOT. YOU ARE NOT ALONE. When we least expect it, God sends company, strength, help, favor...when we least expect. This work of love, this, this caregiving, is a Godly assignment, and God never intended for it to be a solo act, because He is right there with us. Whew, thank goodness; I can release the fear and embrace God's presence and for that, I am grateful.

Graceful Care:

Carefully consider...what may bring about "emotion" so that you can better prepare yourself for it. Sometimes there are things that you just cannot plan.

Avoid perhaps... thinking too long on difficult things; but do what you can to be strong if things get emotional.

Reflect on your feelings...If you find that it is too much, admit it!

This work of love, this, this caregiving, is a Godly assignment, and God never intended for it to be a solo act, because He is right there with us.

Emotional Moments

Until you do, it will be difficult to do something about it.

*E*nrich your experience…When any of this gets to be too much, speak with someone, a counselor, a social worker, a therapist, etc., but do what you can to salvage your mental health! It is important to both you and the person in your care.

Scriptures **to** Ponder

Joshua 1:9 Galatians 5:22-23

CHAPTER 21
Care for the Caregiver

During mid-July of 2020, I became ill. So, what happens when the caregiver needs care? I was managing a schedule that was quite rigorous that summer; I suddenly felt a pounding in my chest, and I realized that I would need medical assistance. In the middle of what I was feeling, so many thoughts went through my mind. *What about Mom? Who is going to take care of her? Will I still be able to care for her after this? Will there be an **after this**?* And, naturally, I was concerned with what was going on with my heart…in the middle of a pandemic!

I ended up in the emergency room, where they basically could not find anything that would cause me to remain hospitalized. In essence, I was sent home because they needed that bed for the *real* sick people. What?! I did not know whether to cry or simply be grateful. So, I followed up with a series of

Care For The Caregiver

tests from my primary care physician, gastroenterologist, and cardiologist, and there were no major heart issues. However, there were some stomach concerns that two prescriptions seemed to manage for now. And what did that have to do with my heart? Even thirty days on a heart monitor did not reveal any major concerns, and I praise God for that. It seemed to me, though, that the doctors may have suspected anxiety. I continued to recover from my medical emergency, receiving help from my husband and son, a friend who checked in almost daily, assisting with household projects, a healthcare provider who helped me with Mom's needs on the weekend, and a niece who literally placed herself on call, along with her son. This unexpected health scare caused me to slow down and reassess my situation. However, the one thing I feel certain of is that my pounding heart was covered by divine intervention, and I am surely convinced of that.

As I reflected on my daily schedule, I really needed to reset my priorities. Four months later, I had an adjusted schedule which included the weekend help for Mom. I knew then that, if I planned to continue caring for her, I would need to pace myself differently. This was my revelation and, at the time, my only earthly solution to my medical conundrum.

I was calmed that evening at the hospital by an indescribable means that I felt only

God's power could provide. I learned a valuable lesson that evening—when caring for someone, self-preservation is key, and planning for personal respite or rest is necessary. This situation was complicated by a worldwide pandemic. Let us face it; I was in no hurry to send Mom anywhere, as the virus was particularly hard on seniors. I was so busy with the daily concerns of Mom's care that I neglected to plan for emergencies on my part. Unfortunately, I did not have a plan in place, and I surely did not have a pandemic plan. The good news was that my village surrounded me with love and helped me through the difficult times, and for that I am grateful to God!

I learned a valuable lesson that evening—when caring for someone, self-preservation is key, and planning for personal respite or rest is necessary.

Graceful Care:

Carefully consider... having a backup plan to provide respite for yourself; your rest time is important.

Avoid perhaps... thinking that you are

superhuman! This act of love must be handled with a huge dose of reality.

Reflect on your feelings…At what point did you decide that no one could do this but you? Be honest! Are you resting? Are you eating? Are you taking good care of yourself? In other words, save yourself from some unnecessary worry by taking a little time to plan for emergencies.

Enrich your experience…create some "if… then" scenarios and think about how you would handle them. For example, ***if*** I could not care for Mom for a day, ***then*** who would I call? This should serve to only make you better prepared in the case of an emergency.

Scriptures **to P**onder

1 Kings 19:7 Psalm 46:1-2 Mark 6:31-32

CHAPTER 22
Just Thankful

As a caregiver, you may experience times when you feel that you are all alone. In the middle of the night, in the quiet of the noonday, or when you seem to have a moment to yourself. Rest assured that you are not. There is a power higher than all of us that keeps us covered with reassurances that we can and will persevere. I have been blessed to have sisters who call to check on Mom, brothers who tend to Mom's business affairs, and nieces and nephews who find their own way of demonstrating that they are genuinely concerned about the well-being of their grandmother (example: moving in with Mom before she moved to Georgia). There are friends and church family who also offer prayers of support and encouragement. I have noted just a few reassurances that the Almighty God sent my way. The names have been eliminated to protect the generosity of the giving heart.

- Sending continuous prayers and well wishes our way
- Calling unexpectedly to say thank you for taking care of Mom
- Offering to foot the bill for Thanksgiving dinner
- Flying in for a day or so to see how things were going
- Sitting with me at the hospital while Mom's needs were addressed (and to be sure I would not have to be admitted)
- Sending funds to help support Mom's care
- Sitting with Mom so that I could enjoy some celebratory moments
- Tending to Mom's business affairs so that I would not have to
- Sending gifts or cards for special occasions (birthdays, Valentine's Day, Mother's Day, Christmas)
- Stopping through on a business or road trip to say hello
- Calling and leaving a message to say, "Hope Mom is doing fine; I know she is because she's in good hands."
- Sending a note of gratitude in the mail
- Being sure I did not need anything or did not want for much

I pray that you can look back on the kind, gentle, and subtle words or actions that have been exhibited as evidence of not being alone. This list is not exhaustive; however, it does attempt to share a gamut of thoughtful gestures to indicate that everyone can do something to offer support! For such acts of kindness, I am so very thankful!

Graceful Care:

Carefully consider…being grateful for discovering the "little things," like cards or calls that mean so much!

Avoid perhaps…thinking any deed is too small.

Reflect on your feelings…Think in terms of gratitude for the kindness that others have shown.

Enrich your experience…with finding all the joy and happiness you can each day; it will benefit the both of you.

I pray that you can look back on the kind, gentle, and subtle words or actions that have been exhibited as evidence of not being alone.

been eliminated to protect the generosity of the giving heart.

- Sending continuous prayers and well wishes our way
- Calling unexpectedly to say thank you for taking care of Mom
- Offering to foot the bill for Thanksgiving dinner
- Flying in for a day or so to see how things were going
- Sitting with me at the hospital while Mom's needs were addressed (and to be sure I would not have to be admitted)
- Sending funds to help support Mom's care
- Sitting with Mom so that I could enjoy some celebratory moments
- Tending to Mom's business affairs so that I would not have to
- Sending gifts or cards for special occasions (birthdays, Valentine's Day, Mother's Day, Christmas)
- Stopping through on a business or road trip to say hello
- Calling and leaving a message to say, "Hope Mom is doing fine; I know she is because she's in good hands."
- Sending a note of gratitude in the mail
- Being sure I did not need anything or did not want for much

I pray that you can look back on the kind, gentle, and subtle words or actions that have been exhibited as evidence of not being alone. This list is not exhaustive; however, it does attempt to share a gamut of thoughtful gestures to indicate that everyone can do something to offer support! For such acts of kindness, I am so very thankful!

Graceful Care:

Carefully consider...being grateful for discovering the "little things," like cards or calls that mean so much!

Avoid perhaps... thinking any deed is too small.

Reflect on your feelings...Think in terms of gratitude for the kindness that others have shown.

Enrich your experience...with finding all the joy and happiness you can each day; it will benefit the both of you.

I pray that you can look back on the kind, gentle, and subtle words or actions that have been exhibited as evidence of not being alone.

Just Thankful

Scriptures **to P**onder

Ephesians 5:20 1 Thessalonians 5:18

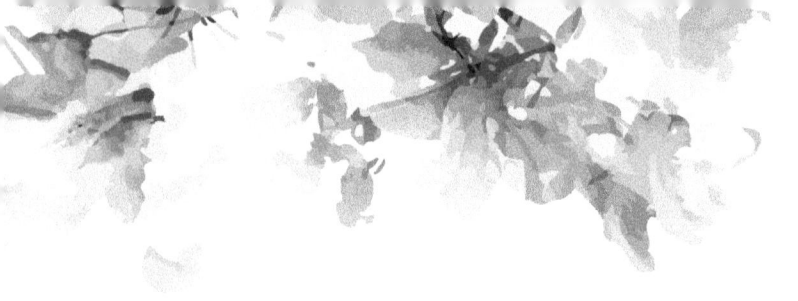

Summary

By now you have probably realized that I am grateful for God's grace and the blessing we have in our matriarch, Ms. Grace. For it is evident to me that I would not have been able to care for Mom without the grace of God; this is my reality. Our home arrangement allowed for the hospice company to visit on a weekly basis and tend to Mom based on their job description. The CNA comes most often, for Mom's daily bath, up to four days per week. This involved talking with Mom while working to ensure that she was comfortable during her bath. The nurse comes once weekly to check her vitals and to order supplies and medications as needed; she also taught me wound care and reported any concerns back to the doctor. The chaplain visited once every two or three weeks to pray, sing, and speak words of encouragement. However, during the viral pandemic, he reached out to me, by call or text, five days a week. Then the social worker takes care of Mom's needs, arranges

Summary

for respite (I call it her "stay-cation"), and surprisingly has great concern for my mental health as well; eventually, I began to understand the importance of that. Initially, I did not welcome the services; however, as time progressed, I learned to appreciate what hospice had to offer.

Hospice companies tout services of care, compassion, and comfort. In many of the workers, I saw more. There was a special dedication to the clients they served. Some of the employees, I think, went beyond the call of duty with things like making sure I had supplies if I unexpectedly ran out; in other words, they made special trips to our home. The way I see it, God was responsible for designing this caregiving assignment. My niece and her family, who cared for Mom in Florida, made the initial contact for the services. Then the process for serving Mom transferred and continued after she came to live with me in Georgia. Once the evaluator came by and explained the services, I reluctantly accepted. I am glad this process was initiated, and I am so grateful to God that a hospice company was available as part of Mom's total care package.

God's grace spans far, wide, and deep. He is the source for all our needs, and I am so thankful that He has shown and continues to show His mercy and grace for Mama Grace, by helping our family care for her. Mom has several wonderful grandchildren who have a special place in her heart. She has two granddaughters who are named after her—Victoria Grace and Brianna Grace, and they too are simply amazing. Writing these reflections has allowed me to look back on the many blessings that God has given and still provides during this journey, since caregiving exudes a willingness to serve from the heart, entrenched in commitment, love, and gratitude.

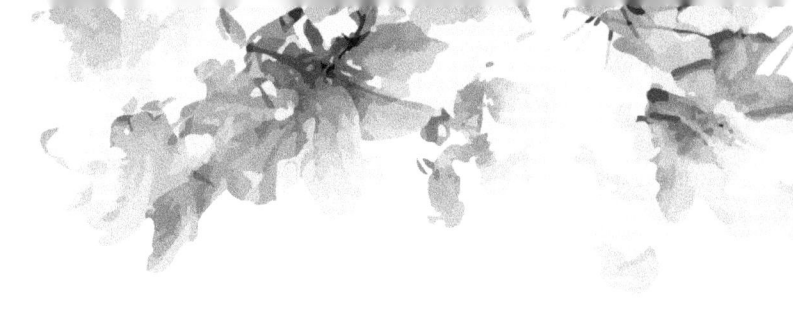

Acknowledgements

My siblings have been amazing in supporting me as I continue to care for our mother. Thank you for the special ways that each of you are sharing in this journey. When I was unable to physically handle Mom, I am so appreciative to my son, and husband for being there during those times for that added "physical support." To my nieces and nephews, that is all the grandchildren that Mom loves so dearly, thank you for the love you have shown to your Grandma Grace. To my church, dance, education, and extended families, I want to thank all of you for taking the time to simply ask about Mom. I also wish to add words of appreciation for all the caregivers and healthcare providers of this world, who are persevering and unselfishly working to keep us safe and well. It means so much to me, and it is my prayer that my gratitude for all of you is reflected in this book.